The Air
Fryer Cookbook for Beginners

Recipes Easy to Make, Fast and Tasty for Frying, Baking and Roasting with Family and Friends

Zera Mallin

TABLE OF CONTENTS

INTRODUCTION	6
BREAKFAST RECIPES	**9**
1. Pork breakfast sticks	9
2. Ww bacon	11
3. Cheese tots	12
BRUNCH RECIPES	**14**
4. Perfect bacon & croissant breakfast	14
5. Ranchero brunch crunch wraps	17
LUNCH RECIPES	**20**
6. Steamed scallops with dill	20
7. Lunch special pancake	22
DINNER RECIPES	**24**
8. Chicken & Turkey Meatloaf	24
9. Turkey Meatballs with Dried Dill	27
10. Chicken Coconut Poppers	29
11. Parmesan Beef Slices	31
DISH RECIPES	**33**
12. Green beans sauté	33
13. Herbed tomatoes	34
14. Coriander potatoes	36
15. Creamy green beans and tomatoes	37
VEGETARIAN RECIPES	**39**
16. Fried Leeks Recipe	39
17. Brussels Sprouts and Tomatoes Mix Recipe	40
18. Radish Hash Recipe	42
19. Broccoli Salad Recipe	43
20. Chili Broccoli	44
21. Parmesan Broccoli and Asparagus	46
22. Butter Broccoli Mix	47

23.	Balsamic Kale	48

POULTRY RECIPES — 50

24.	Curried drumsticks	50
25.	Korean chicken tenders	51
26.	Cholesterol 101 mgHoney lemon chicken wings	52
27.	Air fried chicken with coconut & turmeric	54
28.	Garlic coconut chicken tenders	55

SEAFOOD RECIPES — 57

29.	Sweet cod fillets	57
30.	Pecan cod	59
31.	Balsamic cod	61
32.	Garlic salmon fillets	62
33.	Shrimp and veggie mix	64
34.	White fish with peas and basil	65

MEAT RECIPES — 67

35.	Beef roast	67
36.	Beef tips with onion	69
37.	Buttered rib eye steak	70
38.	Beef jerky	72

DESSERT RECIPES — 75

39.	Baked apple	75
40.	Cinnamon sugar roasted chickpeas	76
41.	Cinnamon fried bananas	77
42.	Brownies	78

APPETIZERS — 81

43.	Chocolate and Hazelnut Cake	81
44.	Jam Tart and Butter-Free Apples	83

SNACKS RECIPES — 86

45.	Pepperoni Chips	86
46.	Crispy Eggplant	87
47.	Steak Nuggets	88

OTHERS RECIPES — 90

48.	Crunchy chicken skin	90
49.	Air fryer pork ribs	92
50.	Air fryer beef tongue	94

LAMB RECIPE 96

51.	BBQ Lamb	96
52.	Lamb Meatballs	97
53.	Glazed Lamb Chops	99
54.	Garlic Lamb Shank	100
55.	Indian Meatball with Lamb	102
56.	Roasted Lamb	104
57.	Lamb Gyro	105
58.	Lemon Lamb Rack	107
59.	Juicy & Savory Lamb Chops	109
60.	Lamb Patties	110

INTRODUCTION

We've put together 50 nutritious recipes that I really love and have tailored to my deep fryer to make you fall in love with air - deep fried food for weight loss wins. Check out these 50 low-carb, nutritious, and easy bake-off-the-air recipes to get you up in the air and looking for food inspiration.

Cooking at home with the assistance of a deep fryer will help you make better decisions if you get enough exercise. There are a variety of excellent ways that air fresheners can assist you with losing weight and being fit.

Changing the way you eat your meals will help you stay on track with your diet and weight loss goals without losing flavor.

Common meals, on the other hand, can be reduced in calories and fat content by substituting air-fried varieties of your preferred ingredients, which can aid weight loss. If you like frying your meals, deep frying in the air is an excellent way to cut calories, minimize fat consumption, and reduce your sensitivity to carcinogens. Switching from deep-frying to air-frying foods, as well as reducing the amount of unhealthy oil consumed on a daily basis, will assist with weight loss.

You risk not consuming a healthy meal if you want to fry canned or frozen foods. If you want fried food but don't want to fry it, make sure your deep fryer recipes just use a small amount of oil. Deep-fryers use less oil, which cuts calories, but you will require 1-2 tablespoons of oil to bake them, which is also more than what is needed for deep-frying.

Make sure you thoroughly choose the ingredients you use in your meals, since not all deep-fryer recipes are safe. Deep fryers can aid in the preparation of healthier foods, but they aren't always safe, so be careful. No matter how much protein you need to lose, weight loss recipes can be made with the right amount of protein.

I often discuss that it's important to avoid excluding tasty foods from one's diet while attempting to lose weight. A slimming menu should include honey-mustard chicken bites, chicken noodles, and chicken fries. While a deep fryer won't do all the work for you, it will assist you in replacing salty, deep-fried foods with nutritious, diet-friendly alternatives. I'll teach you how to make one of my favorite nutritious treats, as well as one of the most amazing fried chicken recipes I've ever had.

Deep fryers are an excellent addition to every kitchen and can help you maintain a balanced diet. Try these low-carb air-fryer recipes if you have a deep fryer and courgettes on hand!

Since you eat less calories on a low-fat diet, you can sustain your weight and avoid weight loss. You will give your diet and weight loss quest a lift by playing with low-calorie meals in the fryer.

It's far cheaper to use a deep fryer instead of a roast since it cuts down on fat and calories without losing flavor. In reality, there are a variety of healthy recipes that can be used as a nutritious substitute for your favorite deep-fried foods. The deep-fried drumsticks are an excellent example of why this kitchen method will help you lose weight and improve your diet. The air cooker is not only simple to use, but it also allows you to behave exactly as you want.

Food cooked in an air fryer has a lower fat and calorie content than food cooked in a deep fryer. In conventional deep-frying, the amount of fat oxidation needed for cooking is much higher than in fried foods. Meals prepared with air frying machines tend to be lower in calories than meals prepared with conventional cooking methods since air frying machines with reduced oil can produce better results.

BREAKFAST RECIPES

1. Pork breakfast sticks

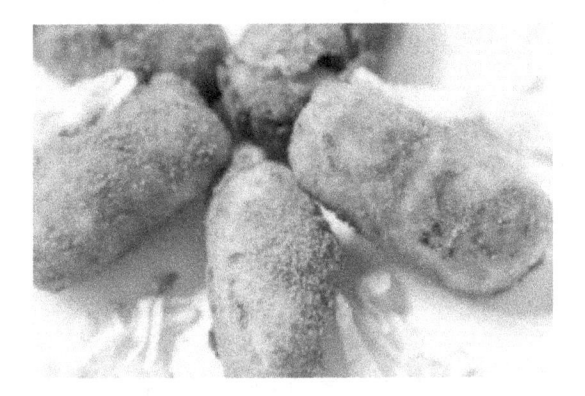

Preparation Time: 15 minutes

Cooking Time: 10 minutes

Servings: 4

Ingredients:

- 1 teaspoon dried basil
- ¼ teaspoon ground ginger
- 1 teaspoon nutmeg
- 1 teaspoon oregano
- 1 teaspoon apple cider vinegar
- 1 teaspoon paprika
- Oz. Pork fillet
- ½ teaspoon salt
- 1 tablespoon olive oil
- 5 oz. Parmesan, shredded

Directions:
1. Cut the pork fillet into thick strips.
2. Then combine the ground ginger, nutmeg, oregano, paprika, and salt in the shallow bowl. Stir it.
3. After this, sprinkle the pork strips with the spice mixture.
4. Sprinkle the meat with the apple cider vinegar.
5. Preheat the air fryer to 380 f.
6. Sprinkle the air fryer basket with the olive oil inside and place the pork strips (sticks) there.
7. Cook the dish for 5 minutes.
8. After this, turn the pork sticks to another side and cook for 4 minutes more.
9. Then cover the pork sticks with the shredded parmesan and cook the dish for 1 minute more.
10. Remove the pork sticks from the air fryer and serve them immediately. The cheese should be soft during the serving.

Nutrition: calories 315, fat 20.4, fiber 0.5, carbs 2.2, protein 31.3

2. Ww bacon

Preparation Time: 8 minutes

Cooking Time: 10 minutes

Servings: 4

Ingredients:

- 8 oz. Bacon
- ½ teaspoon dried oregano
- ½ teaspoon salt
- ½ teaspoon ground black pepper
- ½ teaspoon ground thyme
- 4 oz. Cheddar cheese

Directions:

1. Slice the bacon and rub it with the dried oregano, salt, ground black pepper, and ground thyme from each side.
2. Leave the bacon for 2-3 minutes to make it soak the spices.
3. Meanwhile, preheat the air fryer to 360 f.
4. Place the sliced bacon in the air fryer rack and cook it for 5 minutes.
5. After this, turn the sliced bacon to another side and cook it for 5 minutes more.
6. Meanwhile, shred cheddar cheese.
7. When the bacon is cooked – sprinkle it with the shredded cheese and cook for 30 seconds more.
8. Then transfer the cooked bacon to the plates.

Nutrition: calories 423, fat 33.1, fiber 0.2, carbs 1.5, protein 28.1

3. Cheese tots

Preparation Time: 12 minutes

Cooking Time: 3 minutes

Servings: 5

Ingredients:

- 8 oz. Mozzarella balls
- 1 egg
- ½ cup coconut flakes
- ½ cup almond flour
- 1 teaspoon thyme
- 1 teaspoon ground black pepper
- 1 teaspoon paprika

Directions:

1. Beat the egg in the bowl and whisk it.
2. After this, combine the coconut flour with the thyme, ground black pepper, and paprika. Stir it carefully.
3. Then sprinkle mozzarella balls with the coconut flakes.
4. After this, transfer the balls to the whisked egg mixture.
5. Then coat them in the almond flour mixture.
6. Put mozzarella balls in the freezer for 5 minutes.
7. Meanwhile, preheat the air fryer to 400 f.
8. Put the frozen cheese balls in the preheated air fryer and cook them for 3 minutes.
9. When the time is over – remove the cheese tots from the air fryer basket and chill them for 2 minutes.

Nutrition: calories 166, fat 12.8, fiber 1.4, carbs 2.8, protein 9.5

BRUNCH RECIPES

4. Perfect bacon & croissant breakfast

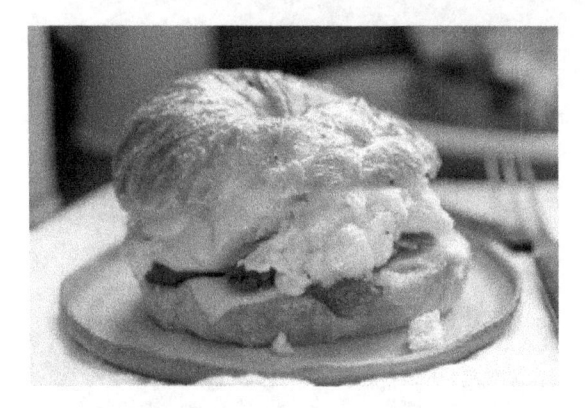

Preparation: 5 minutes

Cooking: 10 minutes

Servings: 2 bacon-croissant sandwiches

Ingredients

- 4 pieces thick-cut bacon
- 2 croissants, sliced
- 2 eggs
- 1 tbsp. Butter
- For the bacon barbecue sauce:
- ½ cup ketchup
- 2 tbsps. Apple cider vinegar
- 1 tbsp. Brown sugar
- 1 tbsp. Molasses
- ½ tbsp. Worcestershire sauce
- ¼ tsp. Onion powder

- ¼ tsp. Mustard powder
- ¼ tsp. Liquid smoke

Directions

1. Preheat your air fryer to 390 degrees f.
2. Meanwhile, incorporate all the barbecue sauce ingredients in a small saucepan. Place the pan over medium heat and bring it to a simmer until the sauce thickens slightly.
3. Place the bacon cuts flat on a tray and brush them with barbecue sauce on one side.
4. Transfer to the air fryer basket with the brushed side up. Cook for about 4-5 minutes then flip the bacon. Brush the other side with bacon sauce and cook for another 5 minutes (or until your desired doneness is achieved).
5. In a medium-size frying pan, melt the butter and fry the eggs according to your preference.
6. Once done, place the eggs at the bottom of each croissant. Top them with two bacon slices each and close with the croissant on top.
7. Serve with your favorite breakfast beverage.

Nutrition: calories – 643; carbohydrates – 57g; fat – 39g; fiber – 1g; protein – 16g; sodium – 1262mg; sugar – 33g

5. Ranchero brunch crunch wraps

Preparation: 5 minutes

Cooking: 15 minutes

Servings: 2 crunch wraps

Ingredients

- 2 servings tofu scramble (or vegan egg)
- 2 large flour tortillas
- 2 small corn tortillas
- ⅓ cup pinto beans, cooked
- ½ cup classic ranchero sauce
- ½ avocado, peeled and sliced
- 2 fresh jalapeños, stemmed and sliced

Directions

1. Assemble the large tortillas on a work surface. Arrange the crunch wraps by stacking the following ingredients in order: tofu or egg scramble, jalapeños, ranchero sauce, corn tortillas, avocado, and pinto beans. You can add more ranchero sauce if desired.
2. Fold the large flour tortilla around the fillings until sealed completely.
3. Place one crunch wrap in the air fryer basket and set the basket on top of the trivet.
4. Air-fry each crunch wrap at 350 degrees f (or 180°c) for 6 minutes. Remove from the basket and transfer to a plate.
5. Repeat step 3 and 4 for the other crunch wrap.

Nutrition: calories – 290; carbohydrates – 26g; fat – 14g; fiber – 11g; protein – 15g; sodium – 340mg; sugar – 3g

LUNCH RECIPES

6. Steamed scallops with dill

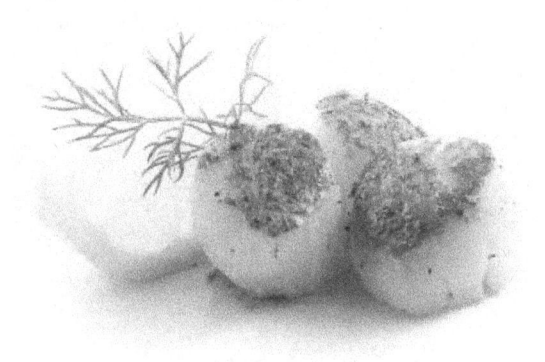

Preparation Time: 5 minutes

Cooking Time: 4 minutes

Servings: 4

Ingredients:

- 1-pound sea scallops
- 1 tablespoon lemon juice
- 2 teaspoons olive oil
- 1 teaspoon dried dill
- Pinch salt
- Freshly ground black pepper

Directions:

1. check the scallops for a small muscle attached to the side and pull it off and discard it.

2. toss the scallops with the lemon juice, olive oil, dill, salt, and pepper. Put into the air fryer basket.
3. steam for 4 to 5 minutes, tossing the basket once during cooking time, until the scallops are just firm when tested with your finger. The internal temperature should be 145°f at minimum.

Nutrition: calories: 121; total fat: 3g; saturated fat: 0g; cholesterol: 37mg; sodium: 223mg; carbohydrates: 3g; fiber: 0g; protein: 19g

7. Lunch special pancake

Preparation Time: 10 minutes

Cooking Time: 10 minutes

Servings: 2

Ingredients:

- 1 tablespoon butter
- 3 eggs, whisked
- ½ cup flour
- ½ cup milk 1 cup salsa
- 1 cup small shrimp, peeled and deveined

Directions:

1. Preheat your air fryer at 400 degrees f, add fryer's pan, add 1 tablespoon butter and melt it.
2. In a bowl, mix eggs with flour and milk, whisk well and pour into air fryer's pan, spread, cook at 350 degrees for 12 minutes and transfer to a plate.
3. In a bowl, mix shrimp with salsa, stir and serve your pancake with this on the side.

Nutrition: calories 200, fat 6, fiber 8, carbs 12, protein 4

DINNER RECIPES

8. Chicken & Turkey Meatloaf

Preparation Time: 15 minutes

Cooking Time: 25 minutes

Servings: 12

Ingredients:

- 3 tbsp. butter
- 10 oz. ground turkey
- 7 oz. ground chicken
- 1 teaspoon dried dill
- ½ tsp ground coriander
- 2 tbsp. almond flour
- 1 tbsp. minced garlic
- 3 oz. fresh spinach
- 1 tsp salt
- 1 egg
- ½ tbsp. paprika
- 1 tsp sesame oil

Directions:

1. Put the ground turkey and ground chicken in a large bowl.
2. Sprinkle the meat with dried dill, ground coriander, almond flour, minced garlic, salt, and paprika. Then chop the fresh spinach and add it to the ground poultry mixture.

3. Crack the egg into the meat mixture and mix well until you get a smooth texture. Get the air fryer basket tray with the olive oil.
4. Preheat the air fryer to 350 F.
5. Roll the ground meat mixture gently to make the flat layer.
6. Put the butter in the center of the meat layer. Make the shape of the meatloaf from the ground meat mixture. Use your fingertips for this step. Place the meatloaf in the air fryer basket tray.
7. Cook for 25 minutes. When the meatloaf is cooked allow it to rest before serving.

Nutrition: Calories 142 Fat 9.8 g Carbs 1.7g Protein 13g

9. Turkey Meatballs with Dried Dill

Preparation Time: 15 minutes

Cooking Time: 11 minutes

Servings: 9

Ingredients:

- 1-pound ground turkey
- 1 tsp chili flakes
- ¼ cup chicken stock
- 2 tbsp. dried dill
- 1 egg
- 1 tsp salt
- 1 tsp paprika
- 1 tbsp. coconut flour
- 2 tbsp. heavy cream
- 1 tsp olive oil

Directions:

1. Crack the egg in a bowl and whisk it with a fork. Add the ground turkey and chili flakes. Sprinkle the mixture with dried dill, salt, paprika, coconut flour, and mix it up. Make the meatballs from the ground turkey mixture. Preheat the air fryer to 360 F.
2. Grease the air fryer basket tray with the olive oil. Then put the meatballs inside. Cook the meatballs for 6 minutes – for 3 minutes on each side.
3. Sprinkle the meatballs with the heavy cream. Cook the meatballs for 5 minutes more. Let them rest for 2-3 minutes when the turkey meatballs are cooked.

Nutrition: Calories124 Fat 7.9g Carbs 1.2g Protein 14.8g

10. Chicken Coconut Poppers

Preparation Time: 10 minutes

Cooking Time: 10 minutes

Servings: 6

Ingredients:

- ½ cup coconut flour
- 1 tsp chili flakes
- 1 tsp ground black pepper
- 1 tsp garlic powder
- 11 oz. chicken breast, boneless, skinless
- 1 tsp olive oil

Directions:

1. Cut the chicken breast into medium cubes and put them in a large bowl. Sprinkle the chicken cubes with the chili flakes, ground black pepper, garlic powder, and stir them well using your hands.
2. After this, sprinkle the chicken cubes with the almond flour.
3. Shake the bowl with the chicken cubes gently to coat the meat.
4. Preheat the air fryer to 365 F.
5. Grease the air fryer basket tray with the olive oil.
6. Place the chicken cubes inside.
7. Cook the chicken poppers for 10 minutes.
8. Turn the chicken poppers over after 5 minutes of cooking.

9. Allow the cooked chicken poppers to cool before serving.

Nutrition: Calories 123, Fat 4.6gCarbs 6.9gProtein 13.2g

11. Parmesan Beef Slices

Preparation Time: 14 minutes

Cooking Time: 25 minutes

Servings: 4

Ingredients:

- 12 oz. beef brisket
- 1 tsp kosher salt
- 7 oz. Parmesan, sliced
- 5 oz. chive stems
- 1 tsp turmeric
- 1 tsp dried oregano
- 2 tsp butter

Directions:

1. Slice the beef brisket into 4 slices.
2. Sprinkle every beef slice with the turmeric and dried oregano.
3. Grease the air fryer basket tray with the butter.
4. Put the beef slices inside.
5. Dice the chives.
6. Make a layer using the diced chives over the beef slices.
7. Then make a layer using the Parmesan cheese.
8. Preheat the air fryer to 365 F.
9. Cook the beef slices for 25 minutes.

Nutrition: Calories 348 Fat 18g Carbs 5g Protein 42.1g

DISH RECIPES

12. Green beans sauté

Preparation Time: 10 minutes

Cooking Time: 20 minutes

Servings: 4

Ingredients:

- 2 pounds green beans, trimmed and halved
- Salt and black pepper to the taste
- 1 tablespoon balsamic vinegar
- 1 tablespoon dill, chopped
- 2 tablespoons olive oil

Directions:

1. In your air fryer's basket, combine the green beans with the vinegar and the other ingredients, toss and cook at 350 degrees f for 20 minutes.
2. Divide between plates and serve as a side dish.

Nutrition: calories 133, fat 3, fiber 8, carbs 16, protein 3

13. Herbed tomatoes

Preparation Time: 10 minutes

Cooking Time: 20 minutes

Servings: 4

Ingredients:

- 1-pound tomatoes, cut into wedges
- 2 tablespoons chives, chopped
- 1 tablespoon oregano, chopped
- 1 tablespoon balsamic vinegar
- 1 teaspoon italian seasoning
- A pinch of salt and black pepper
- 2 tablespoons olive oil

Directions:

1. In your air fryer's basket, combine the tomatoes with the chives, vinegar and the other ingredients, toss and cook at 360 degrees f for 20 minutes.
2. Divide everything between plates and serve as a side dish.

Nutrition: calories 89, fat 7, fiber 9, carbs 4, protein 2

14. Coriander potatoes

Preparation Time: 10 minutes

Cooking Time: 25 minutes

Servings: 4

Ingredients:

- 1-pound gold potatoes, peeled and cut into wedges
- Salt and black pepper to the taste
- 1 tablespoon tomato sauce
- 2 tablespoons coriander, chopped
- ½ teaspoon garlic powder
- 1 teaspoon chili powder
- 1 tablespoon olive oil

Directions:

1. In a bowl, combine the potatoes with the tomato sauce and the other ingredients, toss, and transfer to the air fryer's basket.
2. Cook at 370 degrees f for 25 minutes, divide between plates and serve as a side dish.

Nutrition: calories 210, fat 5, fiber 7, carbs 12, protein 5

15. Creamy green beans and tomatoes

Preparation Time: 10 minutes

Cooking Time: 20 minutes

Servings: 4

Ingredients:

- 1-pound green beans, trimmed and halved
- ½ pound cherry tomatoes, halved
- 2 tablespoons olive oil
- 1 teaspoon oregano, dried
- 1 teaspoon basil, dried
- Salt and black pepper to the taste
- 1 cup heavy cream
- ½ tablespoon cilantro, chopped

Directions:

1. In your air fryer's pan, combine the green beans with the tomatoes and the other ingredients, toss and cook at 360 degrees f for 20 minutes.
2. Divide the mix between plates and serve.

Nutrition: calories 174, fat 5, fiber 7, carbs 11, protein 4

VEGETARIAN RECIPES

16. Fried Leeks Recipe

Preparation Time: 5 minutes

Cooking Time: 10 minutes

Servings: 4

Ingredients:

- 4 leeks; ends cut off and halved
- 1 tbsp. butter; melted
- 1 tbsp. lemon juice
- Salt and black pepper to the taste

Directions:

1. Coat leeks with melted butter, flavor with salt and pepper, put in your air fryer and cook at 350 °F, for 7 minutes.
2. Arrange on a platter, drizzle lemon juice all over and serve

Nutrition: Calories: 100; Fat: 4; Fiber: 2; Carbs: 6; Protein: 2

17. Brussels Sprouts and Tomatoes Mix Recipe

Preparation Time: 5 minutes

Cooking Time: 10 minutes

Servings: 4

Ingredients:

- 1 lb. Brussels sprouts; trimmed
- 6 cherry tomatoes; halved
- 1/4 cup green onions; chopped.
- 1 tbsp. olive oil
- Salt and black pepper to the taste

Directions:

1. Season Brussels sprouts with salt and pepper, put them in your air fryer and cook at 350 °F, for 10 minutes
2. Transfer them to a bowl, add salt, pepper, cherry tomatoes, green onions and olive oil, toss well and serve.

Nutrition: Calories: 121; Fat: 4; Fiber: 4; Carbs: 11; Protein: 4

18. Radish Hash Recipe

Preparation Time: 5 minutes

Cooking Time: 15 minutes

Servings: 4

Ingredients:

- 1/2 tsp. onion powder
- 1/3 cup parmesan; grated
- 4 eggs
- 1 lb. radishes; sliced
- Salt and black pepper to the taste

Directions:

1. In a bowl; mix radishes with salt, pepper, onion, eggs and parmesan and stir well
2. Transfer radishes to a pan that fits your air fryer and cook at 350 °F, for 7 minutes
3. Divide hash on plates and serve.

Nutrition: Calories: 80; Fat: 5; Fiber: 2; Carbs: 5; Protein: 7

19. Broccoli Salad Recipe

Preparation Time: 5 minutes

Cooking Time: 20 minutes

Servings: 4

Ingredients:

- 1 broccoli head; florets separated
- 1 tbsp. Chinese rice wine vinegar
- 1 tbsp. peanut oil
- 6 garlic cloves; minced
- Salt and black pepper to the taste

Directions:

1. In a bowl; mix broccoli with salt, pepper and half of the oil, toss, transfer to your air fryer and cook at 350 °F, for 8 minutes; shaking the fryer halfway
2. Transfer broccoli to a salad bowl, add the rest of the peanut oil, garlic and rice vinegar, toss really well and serve.

Nutrition: Calories: 121; Fat: 3; Fiber: 4; Carbs: 4; Protein: 4

20. Chili Broccoli

Preparation Time: 5 minutes

Cooking Time: 15 minutes

Servings: 4

Ingredients:

- 1-pound broccoli florets
- 2 tablespoons olive oil
- 2 tablespoons chili sauce
- Juice of 1 lime
- A pinch of salt and black pepper

Directions:

1. Combine all of the ingredients in a bowl, and toss well.
2. Put the broccoli in your air fryer's basket and cook at 400 degrees F for 15 minutes.
3. Divide between plates and serve.

Nutrition: Calories 173, Fat 6, Fiber 2, Carbs 6, Protein 8

21. Parmesan Broccoli and Asparagus

Preparation Time: 5 minutes

Cooking Time: 15 minutes

Servings: 4

Ingredients:

- 1 broccoli head, florets separated
- ½ pound asparagus, trimmed
- Juice of 1 lime
- Salt and black pepper to the taste
- 2 tablespoons olive oil
- 3 tablespoons parmesan, grated

Directions:

1. In a small bowl, combine the asparagus with the broccoli and all the other ingredients except the parmesan, toss, transfer to your air fryer's basket and cook at 400 degrees F for 15 minutes.
2. Divide between plates, sprinkle the parmesan on top and serve.

Nutrition: Calories 172, Fat 5, Fiber 2, Carbs 4, Protein 9

22. Butter Broccoli Mix

Preparation Time: 5 minutes

Cooking Time: 15 minutes

Servings: 4

Ingredients:

- 1-pound broccoli florets
- A pinch of salt and black pepper
- 1 teaspoon sweet paprika
- ½ tablespoon butter, melted

Directions:

1. In a small bowl, combine the broccoli with the rest of the ingredients, and toss.
2. Put the broccoli in your air fryer's basket, cook at 350 degrees F for 15 minutes, divide between plates and serve.

Nutrition: Calories 130, Fat 3, Fiber 3, Carbs 4, Protein 8

23. Balsamic Kale

Preparation Time: 2 minutes

Cooking Time: 12 minutes

Servings: 6

Ingredients:

- 2 tablespoons olive oil
- 3 garlic cloves, minced
- 2 and ½ pounds kale leaves
- Salt and black pepper to the taste
- 2 tablespoons balsamic vinegar

Directions:

1. In a pan that fits the air fryer, combine all the ingredients and toss.
2. Put the pan in your air fryer and cook at 300 degrees F for 12 minutes.
3. Divide between plates and serve.

Nutrition: Calories 122, Fat 4, Fiber 3, Carbs 4, Protein 5

POULTRY RECIPES

24. Curried drumsticks

Preparation Time: 10 minutes

Cooking Time: 22 minutes

Servings: 2

Ingredients:

- 2 turkey drumsticks
- 1/3 cup coconut milk
- 1 1/2 tbsp ginger, minced
- 1/4 tsp cayenne pepper
- 2 tbsp red curry paste
- 1/4 tsp pepper
- 1 tsp kosher salt

Directions:

1. Add all ingredients into the bowl and stir to coat. Place in refrigerator for overnight.
2. Spray air fryer basket with cooking spray.
3. Place marinated drumsticks into the air fryer basket and cook at 390 f for 22 minutes.
4. Serve and enjoy.

Nutrition: Calories 279 Fat 18 g Carbohydrates 8 g Sugar 1.5 g Protein 20 g Cholesterol 0 mg

25. Korean chicken tenders

Preparation Time: 10 minutes

Cooking Time: 10 minutes

Servings: 3

Ingredients:

- 12 oz chicken tenders, skinless and boneless
- 2 tbsp green onion, chopped
- 3 garlic cloves, chopped
- 2 tsp sesame seeds, toasted
- 1 tbsp ginger, grated
- 1/4 cup sesame oil
- 1/2 cup soy sauce
- 1/4 tsp pepper

Directions:

1. Slide chicken tenders onto the skewers.
2. In a large bowl, mix together green onion, garlic, sesame seeds, ginger, sesame oil, soy sauce, and pepper.
3. Add chicken skewers into the bowl and coat well with marinade. Place in refrigerator for overnight.
4. Preheat the air fryer to 390 f.
5. Place marinated chicken skewers into the air fryer basket and cook for 10 minutes.

Nutrition: Calories 423 Fat 27 g Carbohydrates 6 g Sugar 1 g Protein 36 g

26. Cholesterol 101 mgHoney lemon chicken wings

Preparation Time: 5 minutes

Cooking Time: 15 minutes

Servings: 8

Ingredients:

- 2 tbsp. Honey
- 2 tbsp. Reduced sodium soy sauce
- 2 tbsp. Freshly squeezed lemon juice
- ½ tsp. Sea salt
- ¼ tsp. White pepper
- ½ tsp. Black pepper
- 16 chicken wings

Directions:

1. In a bowl, mix the honey, soy sauce, lemon juice, salt, white pepper, and black pepper.
2. Soak the chicken wings in the mixture.
3. Cover the bowl and put in the refrigerator for 6 hours.
4. Bring out of the refrigerator.
5. Let sit in room temperature for half an hour.
6. Air fry at 350 degrees f for 6 minutes.
7. Flip over to the other side and cook for another 6 minutes.
8. Flip once more and cook for 3 minutes.

Nutrition: Calories 490 Total fat 19 g Total carbs 8 g Cholesterol 199 mg Sodium 429 mg Potassium 504 mg Protein 71.4 g

27. Air fried chicken with coconut & turmeric

Preparation Time: 5 minutes

Cooking Time: 22 minutes

Servings: 3

Ingredients:

- 1 ½ oz. Coconut milk
- 3 tsp. Ginger, grated
- 4 tsp. Ground turmeric
- ½ tsp. Sea salt
- 3 chicken legs (skin removed)

Directions:

1. Combine the coconut milk, ginger, turmeric and salt.
2. Make a few slits on the chicken meat.
3. Marinate the chicken in the mixture for 4 hours.
4. Keep inside the refrigerator.
5. Preheat air fryer at 375 degrees f.
6. Cook for 10 minutes.
7. Flip and cook for another 10 to 12 minutes.

Nutrition: Calories 112 Total fat 6.5 g Total carbs 4 g Cholesterol 30 mg Sodium 342 mg Potassium 199 mg Protein 9.6 g

28. Garlic coconut chicken tenders

Preparation Time: 10 minutes

Cooking Time: 20 minutes

Servings: 4

Ingredients:

- 2 eggs
- 1 tsp. Sea salt
- ½ tsp. Ground black pepper
- 2 tsp. Garlic powder
- ¾ cup coconut flakes
- ¾ cup panko breadcrumbs
- 1 lb. Chicken tenders (about 8 pieces)

Directions:

1. In a small bowl, beat the eggs and add the salt, black pepper and garlic powder.
2. In another bowl, combine the coconut flakes and breadcrumbs.
3. Dip each of the chicken tenders in the first bowl.
4. Then, dredge with the breadcrumb mixture.
5. Cook the chicken tenders in the air fryer at 375 degrees f for 20 minutes, flipping halfway through.

Nutrition: Calories 242 Total fat 6.7 g Total carbs 16.7 g Cholesterol 140 mg Sodium 520 mg Potassium 377 mg Protein 28.8 g

SEAFOOD RECIPES

29. Sweet cod fillets

Preparation Time: 10 minutes

Cooking Time: 15 minutes

Servings: 4

Ingredients:

- 4 cod fillets, boneless
- Salt and black pepper to taste
- 1 cup water
- 4 tablespoons light soy sauce
- 1 tablespoon sugar
- 3 tablespoons olive oil + a drizzle
- 4 ginger slices
- 3 spring onions, chopped
- 2 tablespoons coriander, chopped

Directions:

1. Season the fish with salt and pepper, then drizzle some oil over it and rub well.
2. Put the fish in your air fryer and cook at 360 degrees f for 12 minutes.
3. Put the water in a pot and heat up over medium heat; add the soy sauce and sugar, stir, bring to a simmer, and remove from the heat.

4. Heat up a pan with the olive oil over medium heat; add the ginger and green onions, stir, cook for 2-3 minutes, and remove from the heat.
5. Divide the fish between plates and top with ginger, coriander, and green onions.
6. Drizzle the soy sauce mixture all over, serve, and enjoy!

Nutrition: calories 270, fat 12, fiber 8, carbs 16, protein 14

30. Pecan cod

Preparation Time: 10 minutes

Cooking Time: 15 minutes

Servings: 2

Ingredients:

- 2 black cod fillets, boneless
- 1 tablespoon olive oil
- Salt and black pepper to taste
- 2 leeks, sliced
- ½ cup pecans, chopped

Directions:

1. In a bowl, mix the cod with the oil, salt, pepper, and the leeks; toss / coat well.
2. Transfer the cod to your air fryer and cook at 360 degrees f for 15 minutes.
3. Divide the fish and leeks between plates, sprinkle the pecans on top, and serve immediately.

Nutrition: calories 280, fat 4, fiber 2, carbs 12, protein 15

31. Balsamic cod

Preparation Time: 5 minutes

Cooking Time: 12 minutes

Servings: 2

Ingredients:

- 2 cod fillets, boneless
- 2 tablespoons lemon juice
- Salt and black pepper to taste
- ½ teaspoon garlic powder
- ⅓ cup water
- ⅓ cup balsamic vinegar
- 3 shallots, chopped
- 2 tablespoons olive oil

Directions:

1. In a bowl, toss the cod with the salt, pepper, lemon juice, garlic powder, water, vinegar, and oil; coat well.
2. Transfer the fish to your air fryer's basket and cook at 360 degrees f for 12 minutes, flipping them halfway.
3. Divide the fish between plates, sprinkle the shallots on top, and serve.

Nutrition: calories 271, fat 12, fiber 10, carbs 16, protein 20

32. Garlic salmon fillets

Preparation Time: 5 minutes

Cooking Time: 8 minutes

Servings: 2

Ingredients:

- 2 salmon fillets, boneless
- Salt and black pepper to taste
- 3 red chili peppers, chopped
- 2 tablespoons lemon juice
- 2 tablespoon olive oil
- 2 tablespoon garlic, minced

Directions:

1. In a bowl, combine the ingredients, toss, and coat fish well.
2. Transfer everything to your air fryer and cook at 365 degrees f for 8 minutes, flipping the fish halfway.
3. Divide between plates and serve right away.

Nutrition: calories 280, fat 4, fiber 8, carbs 15, protein 20

33. Shrimp and veggie mix

Preparation Time: 10 minutes

Cooking Time: 20 minutes

Servings: 4

Ingredients:

- ½ cup red onion, chopped
- 1 cup red bell pepper, chopped
- 1 cup celery, chopped
- 1-pound shrimp, peeled and deveined
- 1 teaspoon worcestershire sauce
- Salt and black pepper to taste
- 1 tablespoon butter, melted
- 1 teaspoon sweet paprika

Directions:

1. Add all the ingredients to a bowl and mix well.
2. Transfer everything to your air fryer and cook 320 degrees f for 20 minutes, shaking halfway.
3. Divide between plates and serve.

Nutrition: calories 220, fat 14, fiber 9, carbs 17, protein 20

34. White fish with peas and basil

Preparation Time: 10 minutes

Cooking Time: 12 minutes

Servings: 4

Ingredients:

- 4 white fish fillets, boneless
- 2 tablespoons cilantro, chopped
- 2 cups peas, cooked and drained
- 4 tablespoons veggie stock
- ½ teaspoon basil, dried
- ½ teaspoon sweet paprika
- 2 garlic cloves, minced
- Salt and pepper to taste

Directions:

1. In a bowl, mix the fish with all ingredients except the peas; toss to coat the fish well.
2. Transfer everything to your air fryer and cook at 360 degrees f for 12 minutes.
3. Add the peas, toss, and divide everything between plates.
4. Serve and enjoy.

Nutrition: calories 241, fat 8, fiber 12, carbs 15, protein 18

MEAT RECIPES

35. Beef roast

Preparation Time: 10 minutes

Cooking Time: 50 minutes

Servings: 6 servings

Ingredients:

- 2½ pounds beef eye of round roast, trimmed
- 2 tablespoons olive oil
- ½ teaspoon onion powder
- ½ teaspoon garlic powder
- ½ teaspoon cayenne pepper
- ½ teaspoon ground black pepper
- Salt, to taste

Directions:

1. In a bowl, mix together the oil, and spices.
2. Generously coat the roast with spice mixture.
3. Set the temperature of air fryer to 360 degrees f. Grease an air fryer basket.
4. Arrange roast into the prepared air fryer basket.
5. Air fry for about 50 minutes.
6. Remove from air fryer and transfer the roast onto a platter.
7. With a piece of foil, cover the roast for about 10 minutes before slicing.
8. Cut the roast into desired size slices and serve.

Nutrition: Calories: 397 Carbohydrate: 0.5g Protein: 55.5g Fat: 12.4g Sugar: 0.2g Sodium: 99mg

36. Beef tips with onion

Preparation Time: 15 minutes

Cooking Time: 10 minutes

Servings: 2 servings

Ingredients:

- 1-pound top round beef, cut into 1½-inch cubes
- ½ yellow onion, chopped
- 2 tablespoons worcestershire sauce
- 1 tablespoon avocado oil
- 1 teaspoon onion powder
- 1 teaspoon garlic powder
- Salt and ground black pepper, as required

Directions:

1. In a bowl, mix together the beef tips, onion, worcestershire sauce, oil, and spices.
2. Set the temperature of air fryer to 360 degrees f. Grease an air fryer basket.
3. Arrange beef mixture into the prepared air fryer basket.
4. Air fry for about 8-10 minutes.
5. Remove from air fryer and transfer the steak mixture onto serving plates.
6. Serve hot.

Nutrition: Calories: 266 Carbohydrate: 4g Protein: 36.3g Fat: 10.5g Sugar: 2.5g Sodium: 192mg

37. Buttered rib eye steak

Preparation Time: 20 minutes

Cooking Time: 14 minutes

Servings: 2 servings

Ingredients:

- ½ cup unsalted butter, softened
- 2 tablespoons fresh parsley, chopped
- 2 teaspoons garlic, minced
- 1 teaspoon worcestershire sauce
- Salt, as required
- 2 (8-ounces) rib eye steak
- Ground black pepper, as required
- 1 tablespoon olive oil

Directions:

1. In a bowl, add the butter, parsley, garlic, worcestershire sauce, and salt. Mix until well combined.
2. Place the butter mixture onto a parchment paper and roll into a log.
3. Refrigerate until using.
4. Coat the steak evenly with oil and then, sprinkle with salt and black pepper.
5. Set the temperature of air fryer to 400 degrees f. Grease an air fryer basket.
6. Arrange steaks into the prepared air fryer basket.
7. Air fry for about 14 minutes, flipping once halfway through.

8. Remove from air fryer and place the steaks onto a platter for about 5 minutes.
9. Cut each steak into desired size slices and divide onto serving plates.
10. now, cut the butter log into slices.
11. top each steak with butter slices and serve.

Nutrition: Calories: 731 Carbohydrate: 1.2g Protein: 27.3g Fat: 68.8g Sugar: 0.4g Sodium: 375mg

38. Beef jerky

Preparation Time: 20 minutes

Cooking Time: 1 hour

Servings: 3 servings

Ingredients:

- ½ cup dark brown sugar
- ½ cup soy sauce
- ¼ cup worcestershire sauce
- 1 tablespoon chili pepper sauce
- 1 tablespoon hickory liquid smoke
- 1 teaspoon garlic powder
- 1 teaspoon onion powder
- 1 teaspoon cayenne pepper
- ½ teaspoon smoked paprika
- ½ teaspoon ground black pepper
- 1-pound bottom round beef, cut into thin strips

Directions:

1. In a large bowl, mix together the brown sugar, all sauces, liquid smoke, and spices.
2. Add the beef strips and generously coat with marinade.
3. Cover the bowl and marinate overnight.
4. Set the temperature of air fryer to 180 degrees f. Lightly, grease an air fryer basket.
5. Remove the beef strips from fridge and with paper towels, pat them dry.
6. Arrange half of the beef strips in the bottom of prepared air fryer basket in a single layer.

7. Now, arrange a cooking rack over the strips.
8. Place the remaining beef strips on top of the rack in a single layer.
9. Air fry for about 1 hour.
10. Remove from air fryer and arrange the strips onto a paper towel-lined baking sheet to cool completely before serving.

Nutrition: Calories: 471 Carbohydrate: 33.1g Protein: 48.7g Fat: 14.8g Sugar: 28.8g Sodium: 2000mg

DESSERT RECIPES

39. Baked apple

Preparation Time: 10 minutes

Cooking Time: 20 minutes

Servings: 4

Ingredients:

- ¼ c. Water
- ¼ tsp. Nutmeg
- ¼ tsp. Cinnamon
- 1 ½ tsp. Melted ghee
- 2 tbsp. Raisins
- 2 tbsp. Chopped walnuts
- 1 medium apple

Directions:

1. Preheat your air fryer to 350 degrees.
2. Slice apple in half and discard some of the flesh from the center.
3. Place into frying pan.
4. Mix remaining ingredients together except water. Spoon mixture to the middle of apple halves.
5. Pour water over filled apples.
6. Place pan with apple halves into air fryer, bake 20 minutes.

Nutrition: Calories: 199 fat: 9g protein: 1g sugar: 3g

40. Cinnamon sugar roasted chickpeas

Preparation Time: 10 minutes

Cooking Time: 10 minutes

Servings: 2

Ingredients:

- 1 tbsp. Sweetener
- 1 tbsp. Cinnamon
- 1 c. Chickpeas

Directions:

1. Preheat air fryer to 390 degrees.
2. Rinse and drain chickpeas.
3. Mix all ingredients together and add to air fryer.
4. Cook 10 minutes.

Nutrition: Calories: 111 fat: 19g protein: 16g sugar: 5g

41. Cinnamon fried bananas

Preparation Time: 5 minutes

Cooking Time: 10 minutes

Servings: 2-3

Ingredients:

- 1 c. Panko breadcrumbs
- 3 tbsp. Cinnamon
- ½ c. Almond flour
- 3 egg whites
- 8 ripe bananas
- 3 tbsp. Vegan coconut oil

Directions:

1. Heat coconut oil and add breadcrumbs. Mix around 2-3 minutes until golden. Pour into bowl.
2. Peel and cut bananas in half. Roll each bananas half into flour, eggs, and crumb mixture. Place into air fryer.
3. Cook 10 minutes at 280 degrees.
4. A great addition to a healthy banana split!

Nutrition: Calories: 219 fat: 10g protein: 3g sugar: 5g

42. Brownies

Preparation Time: 5 minutes

Cooking Time: 20 minutes

Servings: 4

Ingredients:

- The wet **ingredients:**
- 1/4 cup almond milk
- 1/4 cup chickpeas liquid
- 1/2 teaspoon vanilla extract, unsweetened
- The dry **ingredients:**
- 1/2 cup whole-wheat pastry flour
- 1/2 cup coconut sugar
- 1/4 cup cocoa powder, unsweetened
- 1 tablespoon ground flax seeds
- 1/4 teaspoon salt
- For the mix-ins:
- 2 tablespoons chopped walnuts
- 2 tablespoons pecans
- 2 tablespoons shredded coconut

Directions:

1. Switch on the air fryer, insert the fryer basket, then shut it with the lid, set the frying temperature 350 degrees f, and let it preheat for 5 minutes.
2. Meanwhile, take a large bowl, add all the dry ingredients in it and stir until mixed.
3. Take another bowl, place all the wet ingredients in it, whisk until combined, then gradually mix into the dry

ingredients mixture until incorporated and mix the walnuts, pecans and coconut until combined.
4. Take a 5-inch round pan, line it with parchment paper, pour in prepared batter, smooth the top with a spatula.
5. Open the preheated fryer, place the prepared pan in it, close the lid and cook for 20 minutes until firm and a toothpick come out clean from the center of the pan.
6. When done, the air fryer will beep, then open the lid, remove the pan from the fryer and cool for 15 minutes.
7. Then cut into brownies and serve.

Nutrition: Calories: 262 cal Fat: 9.9 g Carbs: 47.9 g Protein: 3.2 g Fiber: 4.8 g

APPETIZERS

43. Chocolate and Hazelnut Cake

Preparation Time: 10 minutes

Cooking Time: 25 minutes

Servings: 22

Ingredients:

- 3 eggs
- 100 g caster sugar
- 220 g flour
- 30 g bitter cocoa
- 50 ml lactose-free milk
- 40 ml Seed oil
- 1 sachet Baking powder
- 80 g whole hazelnuts

Directions:

1. Whip the eggs with the sugar with the electric whisk for a few minutes until foamy.
2. Add the milk and oil flush, mixing with low speed electric whisk. Then add the flour and the bitter cocoa by sieving them.
3. When the mixture is fluid, also add the baking powder. The dough is ready.
4. Pour the dough into a 22 cm diameter cake mold that enters the air fryer basket. Level it well.

5. Add the whole toasted hazelnuts to the surface, just chopped.
6. Cook in an air fryer at 160 ° for 15 minutes and then at 180 ° for another 10 minutes. Always check with a toothpick after at least 20 minutes. If it still seems undercooked, continue for a few minutes.
7. Bake in a preheated oven at 180 ° in static mode for about 40 minutes, always making the toothpick test.

Nutrition: Calories: 453; Fat: 14g; Protein: 29g; Fiber: 14g

44. Jam Tart and Butter-Free Apples

Preparation Time: 15 minutes

Cooking Time: 20 minutes

Servings: 20-22

Ingredients:

- For the Oil Shortbread:
- 300 g flour 00
- 100 g caster sugar
- 2 eggs
- 70 ml Seed oil (corn or sunflower)
- 1 teaspoon baking powder
- For the stuffing
- 120 g cherry jam
- 2 red apples

Directions:

1. Prepare the short crust pastry without butter following this recipe. You can also use it immediately; it does not require rest.
2. Then, spread the pastry on the lightly floured work surface and prepare a sheet of about half a centimeter. Leave some for the strips.
3. Turn it upside down on the tart mold of 20-22 cm depending on the size of the basket of your air fryer.
4. use a perforated mold with removable bottom: in this way the air can circulate more easily and cook the tart faster.

5. Spread the jam and level it well. Peel the apples, remove the core and cut them into slices.
6. Spread the apples in rays on the jam. With the remaining short crust pastry cut out strips with a smooth or toothed wheel.
7. Place the strips on the tart and cook.
8. Place the mold directly on the basket and operate it at 160 ° or with the cake function.
9. Cook for 15 minutes and then another 5 minutes at 180 ° until golden brown, even on the bottom.
10. Bake in a preheated oven at 180 ° in static mode for about 40 minutes until golden brown, in the central shelf.
11. Let it cool well before removing it from the mold.
12. You can keep it for a maximum week wrapped in aluminum foil.

Nutrition: Calories: 567; Fat:22g; Protein:38g; Fiber:15g

SNACKS RECIPES

45. Pepperoni Chips

Preparation Time: 2 minutes

Cooking Time: 8 minutes

Servings: 6

Ingredients:

- 6 oz. pepperoni slices

Directions:

1. Place one batch of pepperoni slices in the air fryer basket.
2. Cook for 8 minutes at 360 F.
3. Cook remaining pepperoni slices using same steps.
4. Serve and enjoy.

Nutrition: Calories 51 Fat 1 g Carbohydrates 2 g Sugar 1.3 g Protein 0 g Cholesterol 0 mg

46. Crispy Eggplant

Preparation Time: 5 minutes

Cooking Time: 20 minutes

Servings: 4

Ingredients:

- 1 eggplant, cut into 1-inch pieces
- 1/2 tsp Italian seasoning
- 1 tsp paprika
- 1/2 tsp red pepper
- 1 tsp garlic powder
- 2 tbsp. olive oil

Directions:

1. Add all ingredients into the large mixing bowl and toss well.
2. Transfer eggplant mixture into the air fryer basket.
3. Cook at 375 F for 20 minutes. Shake basket halfway through.
4. Serve and enjoy.

Nutrition: Calories 99 Fat 7.5 g Carbohydrates 8.7 g Sugar 4.5 g Protein 1.5 g Cholesterol 0 mg

47. Steak Nuggets

Preparation Time: 10 minutes

Cooking Time: 15 minutes

Servings: 4

Ingredients:

- 1 lb. beef steak, cut into chunks
- 1 large egg, lightly beaten
- 1/2 cup pork rind, crushed
- 1/2 cup parmesan cheese, grated
- 1/2 tsp salt

Directions:

1. Add egg in a small bowl.
2. In a shallow bowl, mix together pork rind, cheese, and salt.
3. Dip each steak chunk in egg then coat with pork rind mixture and place on a plate. Place in refrigerator for 30 minutes.
4. Spray air fryer basket with cooking spray.
5. Preheat the air fryer to 400 F.
6. Place steak nuggets in air fryer basket and cook for 15-18 minutes or until cooked. Shake after every 4 minutes.
7. Serve and enjoy.

Nutrition: Calories 609 Fat 38 g Carbohydrates 2 g Sugar 0.4 g Protein 63 g Cholesterol 195 mg

OTHERS RECIPES

48. Crunchy chicken skin

Preparation Time: 10 minutes

Cooking Time: 6 minutes

Servings: 6

Ingredients:

- 1-pound chicken skin
- 1 teaspoon dried dill
- ½ teaspoon ground black pepper
- ½ teaspoon chili flakes
- ½ teaspoon salt
- 1 teaspoon butter

Directions:

1. Slice the chicken skin roughly and sprinkle it with the dried dill, ground black pepper, chili flakes, and salt.
2. Mix the chicken skin up.
3. Melt the butter and add it to the chicken skin mixture.
4. Mix the chicken skin with the help of the spoon.
5. Then preheat the air fryer to 360 f.
6. Put the prepared chicken skin in the air fryer basket.
7. Cook the chicken skin for 3 minutes from each side. Cook the chicken skin more if you want the crunchy effect.
8. Transfer the cooked chicken skin in the paper towel and let it dry.

9. Then serve the chicken skin.

Nutrition: calories 350, fat 31.4, fiber 0.1, carbs 0.2, protein 15.5

49. Air fryer pork ribs

Preparation Time: 30 minutes

Cooking Time: 30 minutes

Servings: 5

Ingredients:

- 1 tablespoon apple cider vinegar
- 1 teaspoon cayenne pepper
- 1 teaspoon minced garlic
- 1 teaspoon mustard
- 1 teaspoon chili flakes
- 16 oz. Pork ribs
- 1 teaspoon sesame oil
- 1 teaspoon salt
- 1 tablespoon paprika

Directions:

1. Chop the pork ribs roughly.
2. Then sprinkle the pork ribs with the cayenne pepper, apple cider vinegar, minced garlic, mustard, and chili flakes.
3. Then add the sesame oil and salt.
4. Add paprika and mix the pork ribs carefully.
5. Leave the pork ribs in the fridge for 20 minutes.
6. After this, preheat the air fryer to 360 f.
7. Transfer the pork ribs in the air fryer basket and cook them for 15 minutes.
8. After this, turn the pork ribs to another side and cook the meat for 15 minutes more.

9. Then transfer the pork ribs in the serving bowls.

Nutrition: calories 265, fat 17.4, fiber 0.7, carbs 1.4, protein 24.5

50. Air fryer beef tongue

Preparation Time: 10 minutes

Cooking Time: 20 minutes

Servings: 6

Ingredients:

- 1-pound beef tongue
- 1 teaspoon salt
- 1 teaspoon ground black pepper
- 1 teaspoon paprika
- 1 tablespoon butter
- 4 cup water

Directions:

1. Preheat the air fryer to 365 f.
2. Put the beef tongue in the air fryer basket tray and add water.
3. Sprinkle the mixture with the salt, ground black pepper, and paprika.
4. Cook the beef tongue for 15 minutes.
5. After this, strain the water from the beef tongue.
6. Cut the beef tongue into the strips.
7. Then toss the butter in the air fryer basket tray and add the beef strips.
8. Cook the beef tongue strips for 5 minutes at 360 f.
9. When the beef tongue is cooked – transfer the dish to the serving plate.

Nutrition: calories 234, fat 18.8, fiber 0.2, carbs 0.4, protein 14.7

LAMB RECIPE

51. **BBQ Lamb**

Preapration Time: 90 minutes

Cooking Time: 15 minutes

Servings: 8

Ingredients:
- 4 lbs boneless leg of lamb, cut into 2-inch chunks
- 2-1/2 tbsps herb salt
- 2 tbsps olive oil

Directions:
1. Preheat the PowerXL Air Fryer Grill by selecting air fryer mode
2. Adjust the temperature to 390°F, set Time to 5 minutes
3. Season the meat with salt and olive oil
4. Arrange on the Air fryer baking tray
5. Transfer to the PowerXL Air Fryer Grill
6. Air fry for 15 minutes, flipping halfway through
7. Serve and enjoy
8. Serving Suggestions: serve with marinara sauce
9. Directions: & Cooking Tips: work in batches

Nutrition: Calories: 341kcal, Fat: 16g, Carb: 1g, Proteins: 26g

52. Lamb Meatballs

Preapration Time: 15minutes

Cooking Time: 15 minutes

Servings: 12

Ingredients:
- 1 lb. ground lamb
- 1/2 cup breadcrumbs
- 1 lemon, juiced and zested
- 1/4 cup milk
- 2 egg yolks
- 1 tsp ground cumin
- 1 tsp dried oregano
- 1/2 tsp salt
- 1 tsp ground coriander
- 1/2 tsp black pepper
- 3 garlic cloves, minced
- 1/4 cup fresh parsley, chopped
- 1/2 cup crumbled feta cheese

Directions:
1. Preheat the PowerXL Air Fryer Grill by selecting Broil mode
2. Adjust the temperature to 390°F, set Time to 5 minutes
3. Combine all the Ingredients:in a bowl
4. Form into 12 balls
5. Arrange on the Air fryer baking tray
6. Transfer to the PowerXL Air Fryer Grill
7. Cook for 12 minutes
8. Serve and enjoy
9. Serving Suggestions: Serve with tzatziki sauce

10. Directions: & Cooking Tips: rub olive oil on your hand when forming the meatballs

Nutrition: Calories: 129kcal, Fat: 6.4g, Carb: 4.9g, Proteins: 25g

53. Glazed Lamb Chops

Preapration Time: 30 minutes
Cooking Time: 15 minutes
Servings: 4

Ingredients:
- 4 (4-ounce) lamb loin chops
- 1 tbsp Dijon mustard
- 1 tsp honey
- 1/2 tbsp fresh lime juice
- 1/2 tsp olive oil
- Salt and ground black pepper, as required

Directions:
1. Preheat the PowerXL Air Fryer Grill by selecting air fryer mode
2. Adjust the temperature to 3900 F, set Time to 5 minutes
3. Combine all the Ingredients:in a bowl
4. Add the pork chops and toss to coat
5. Arrange on the Air fryer baking tray
6. Transfer to the PowerXL Air Fryer Grill
7. Air fry for 15 minutes, flipping halfway through
8. Serve and enjoy
9. Serving Suggestions: Serve while still hot
10. Directions: & Cooking Tips: leave to marinate for a few minutes

Nutrition: Calories: 224kcal, Fat: 4g, Carb: 2g, Proteins: 19g

54. Garlic Lamb Shank

Preapration Time: 15 minutes
Cooking Time: 24 minutes
Servings: 4

Ingredients:
- 17 oz. lamb shanks
- 2 tbsp garlic, peeled and coarsely chopped
- tsp kosher salt
- 1/2 cup chicken stock
- tbsp dried parsley
- 1 tsp dried rosemary
- 4 oz. chive stems, chopped
- 1 tsp butter
- 1 tsp nutmeg
- 1/2 tsp ground black pepper

Directions:
1. Make the cuts in the lamb shank and fill the cuts with the chopped garlic.
2. Sprinkle the lamb shank with the kosher salt, dried parsley, dried rosemary, nutmeg, and ground black pepper.
3. Stir the spices on the lamb shank gently.
4. Preheat the PowerXL Air Fryer Grill by selecting air fry mode.
5. Adjust the temperature to 380°F, set Time to 5 minutes
6. put the butter, chives, and chicken stock in the air fryer baking tray.
7. Add the lamb shank and air fry the meat for 24 minutes.
8. Serve and enjoy
9. Serving Suggestions: Serve with the cooking liquid
10. Directions: & Cooking Tips: add spices to taste

Nutrition: Calories: 205kcal, Fat: 8.2g, Carb: 3g, Proteins: 28g

55. Indian Meatball with Lamb

Preapration Time: 10 minutes

Cooking Time: 14minutes

Servings: 8

Ingredients:
- 1 lb. ground lamb
- 1 garlic clove, minced
- 1 egg
- 1 tbsp butter
- 4 oz. chive stems, grated
- 1/4 tbsp turmeric
- 1/3 tsp cayenne pepper
- 1/4 tsp bay leaf
- 1 tsp ground coriander
- 1 tsp salt
- 1 tsp ground black pepper

Directions:
1. Combine all the Ingredients:together in a bowl
2. Preheat the PowerXL air fryer by selecting the air fry mode
3. Adjust the temperature to 390°F and set Time to 5 minutes
4. Put the butter in the Air fryer baking tray and melt it.
5. Form the meatballs
6. Place them in the air fryer baking tray.
7. Transfer to the PowerXL Air Fryer Grill
8. Cook the dish for 14 minutes.
9. Stir the meatballs twice during the cooking
10. Serving Suggestions: Serve with salad and sauce
11. Directions: & Cooking Tips: use an ice-cream scooper to form the balls

Nutrition: Calories: 300kcal, Fat: 13g, Carb: 19g, Proteins: 21g

56. Roasted Lamb

Preapration Time: 60 minutes

Cooking Time: 13 minutes

Servings: 4

Ingredients:
- 2-1/2 pounds lamb leg roast, slits carved
- tbsp olive oil
- garlic cloves, sliced into smaller slithers
- 1 tbsp dried rosemary
- Cracked Himalayan rock salt and cracked peppercorns, to taste

Directions:
1. Make the cuts in the lamb roast and insert them with garlic.
2. Sprinkle the lamb roast with kosher salt, rosemary, and ground black pepper.
3. Brush with oil.
4. Preheat the PowerXL Air Fryer Grill by selecting air fry mode.
5. Adjust the temperature to 380°F, set Time to 5 minutes
6. Place the lamb roast on the Baking Pan
7. Transfer to the PowerXL Air Fryer Grill.
8. Air fry for 1 hour 15 minutes
9. Serve and enjoy
10. Serving Suggestions: serve with mushroom sauce
11. Directions: & Cooking Tips: leave to marinate for some minutes

Nutrition: Calories: 246kcal, Fat: 7g, Carb: 9g, Proteins: 33g

57. Lamb Gyro

Preapration Time: 20 minutes
Cooking Time: 15 minutes
Servings: 4

Ingredients:
- 1 pound ground lamb
- 1/2 onion sliced
- 1/4 cup mint, minced
- 1/4 red onion, minced
- 1/8 tsp rosemary
- 1/2 tsp salt
- 1/2 tsp black pepper
- 3/4 cup hummus
- 4 slices pita bread
- 1/2 cucumber, peeled and sliced into thin rounds
- 1 cup romaine lettuce, shredded
- 1 Roma tomato, diced
- 1/4 cup parsley, minced
- 2 cloves garlic, minced
- 12 mint leaves, minced

Directions:
1. Preheat the PowerXL Air Fryer Grill by selecting broil mode
2. Adjust the temperature to 3700F, set Time to 5 minutes
3. Mix lamb with onions, mint, parsley, garlic, salt, rosemary, and pepper
4. Form into patties
5. Arrange in a lined Air fryer baking tray
6. Transfer to the PowerXL Air Fryer Grill
7. Air fry for 20 minutes, flipping halfway through

8. Assemble the gyro with the remaining Ingredients:
9. Serve and enjoy
10. Serving Suggestions: serve drizzled with tzatziki sauce
11. Directions: & Cooking Tips: mix until well incorporated

Nutrition:Calories: 309kcal, Fat: 14.6g, Carb: 29g, Proteins: 19g

58. Lemon Lamb Rack

Preapration Time: 30 minutes

Cooking Time: 10 minutes

Servings: 4

Ingredients:
- 1/4 cup olive oil
- 3 tbsp garlic, minced
- 1/3 cup dry white wine
- 1 tbsp lemon zest, grated
- 2 tbsps lemon juice
- 1-1/2 tsp dried oregano, crushed
- 1 tsp thyme leaves, minced
- Salt and black pepper
- 4 lamb rack
- 1 lemon, sliced

Directions:
1. Whisk everything in a baking pan to coat the chicken breasts well.
2. Place the lemon slices on top of the chicken breasts.
3. Spread the mustard mixture over the toasted bread slices.
4. Press "Power Button" of Air Fry Oven and turn the dial to select the "Bake" mode.
5. Press the Time button and again turn the dial to set the cooking Time to 30 minutes.
6. Now push the Temp button and rotate the dial to set the temperature at 370 degrees F.
7. Once preheated, place the baking pan inside and close its lid.
8. Serve warm.

9. Preheat the PowerXL Air Fryer Grill by selecting air fryer mode
10. Adjust the temperature to 3700F, set Time to 5 minutes
11. Whisk all the Ingredients:together in a bowl
12. Pour into air fryer baking tray
13. Add the lamb rack
14. Top with lemon
15. Transfer to the PowerXL Air Fryer Grill
16. Air fry for 30 minutes, flipping halfway through
17. Serve and enjoy
18. Serving Suggestions: Serve with the juice
19. Directions: & Cooking Tips: Leave to marinate for a few minutes

Nutrition: Calories: 288kcal, Fat: 7g, Carb: 5g, Proteins: 16g

59. Juicy & Savory Lamb Chops

Preapration Time:10 minutes

Cooking Time: 10 minutes

Servings:1

Ingredients:
- 1/3 lb lamb chop
- 1 tbsp mixed fresh herbs, chopped
- 1/2 tbsp olive oil
- 1/2 tbsp Dijon mustard
- Pepper
- Salt

Directions:
1. Season lamb chop with pepper and salt.
2. In a small bowl, mix together oil, mustard, and mixed herbs.
3. Brush lamb chop from both the sides with oil mixture.
4. Place lamb chop into the air fryer basket and cook at 375 F for 10 minutes. Turn halfway through.

Nutrition: Calories 350 Fat 18.5 g Carbohydrates 1.2 g Sugar 0.1 g Protein 43 g Cholesterol 136 mg

60. Lamb Patties

Preapration Time:10 minutes
Cooking Time: 30 minutes
Servings:4

Ingredients:
- 1 lb ground lamb meat
- 1 egg, lightly beaten
- 1/2 tbsp garlic, minced
- 1 spring onion, chopped
- 1/4 cup almond flour
- 1 tbsp basil, chopped
- 1 tbsp cilantro, chopped
- Pepper
- Salt

Directions:
1. Spray air fryer basket with cooking spray.
2. Add all Ingredients:into the bowl and mix until well combined.
3. Make small patties from meat mixture and place into the air fryer basket and cook at 390 F for 30 minutes. Turn patties halfway through.
4. Serve and enjoy.

Nutrition: Calories 260 Fat 17 g Carbohydrates 1.1 g Sugar 0.2 g Protein 23 g Cholesterol 121 mg

CPSIA information can be obtained
at www.ICGtesting.com
Printed in the USA
BVHW062108150621
609639BV00003B/679